Herbs for Health and Healing

The Healing Power of 10 Herbs, Spices, and Healing Plants

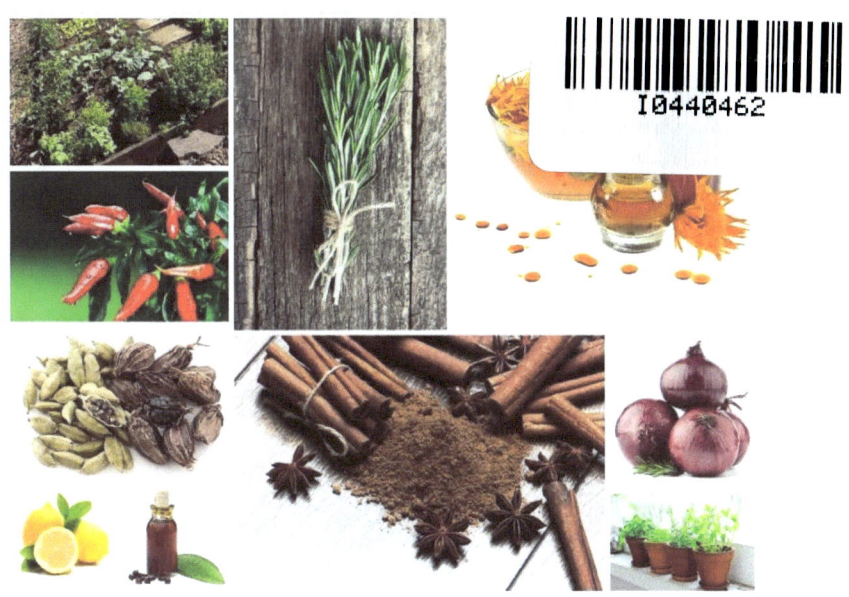

Dueep Jyot Singh

Health Learning Series

Mendon Cottage Books

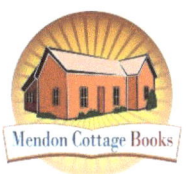

JD-Biz Publishing

Disclaimer

The information is this book is provided for informational purposes only. It is not intended to be used and medical advice or a substitute for proper medical treatment by a qualified health care provider. The information is believed to be accurate as presented based on research by the author.

The contents have not been evaluated by the U.S. Food and Drug Administration or any other Government or Health Organization and the contents in this book are not to be used to treat cure or prevent disease.

The author or publisher is not responsible for the use or safety of any diet, procedure or treatment mentioned in this book. The author or publisher is not responsible for errors or omissions that may exist.

Warning

The Book is for informational purposes only and before taking on any diet, treatment or medical procedure, it is recommended to consult with your primary health care provider.

Our books are available at

1. Amazon.com
2. Barnes and Noble
3. Itunes
4. Kobo
5. Smashwords
6. Google Play Books

Table of Contents

Introduction

This 21st century world is full of toxic water, poisoned air, and chemical pollution. We are also very worried about the thinning ozone layer, because it is definitely going to have a bad after effect on our climate, and then correspondingly on our health.

This is the reason why, we are looking towards the use of natural elements, to keep us healthy and fit. That is because we have understood the fact that chemical-based drugs are efficacious on a short-term basis, but they do not heal us long-term. Besides, there is always the chance of dangerous side effects. And so our health is ruined, because we could not prevent ourselves from popping that pill.

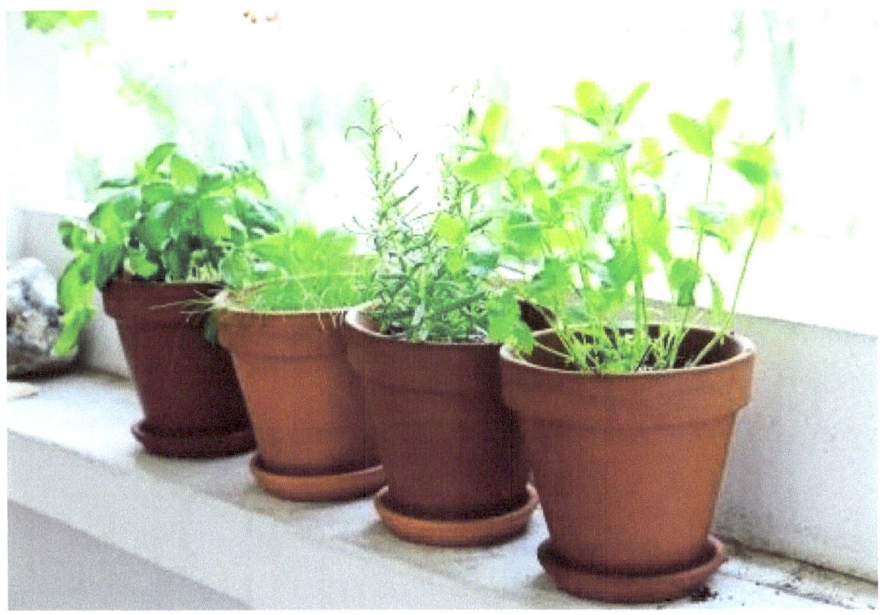

Ancient remedies, on the other hand, have been passed down through centuries. Many of us consider these remedies to be quack remedies, because many of them have not been subjected to scientific research, and a stamp of experienced researchers telling you, all right, it is useful to add a lot of cinnamon to your diet, because that has been scientifically proven to cure 99% of bacterial and viral infections.

Nevertheless, there are a lot of infections, which have been proven down the millenniums to be cured only by practical and natural remedies. Many of these practical remedies have been in use for thousands of years and are still in use because they have proved their time tested efficacy over and over again in solving your health problems and curing you. Best, you are going to be cured from the root, and the effects are going to be long-term.

No matter what ailment you suffer from, you can always do something with a little bit of knowledge, and a little bit of help from nature to enhance your well-being and good health.

Many of us living in the cities are terrified of picking up any useful herbal plant material growing wild and which we encounter when we are on open-air ambles, because we know that they have been contaminated from lead from vehicle exhausts, and also could have been sprayed with agri-chemicals. Also, we do not have the herbal lore, which was taught to our ancestors, by their ancestors. There was a time when every proud housewife worth her salt knew all about herbs, spices and natural remedies and had a stillroom in which she used to brew herbal remedies to keep our family healthy and happy, and natural ointments to keep them youthful looking.

Gathering herbs from the wild can only be done by those botanists and herbalists will have extensive knowledge of the beneficial points of plants.

So that is the reason why a large number of the plants which I am going to describe to you in this book can be easily found in your local market.

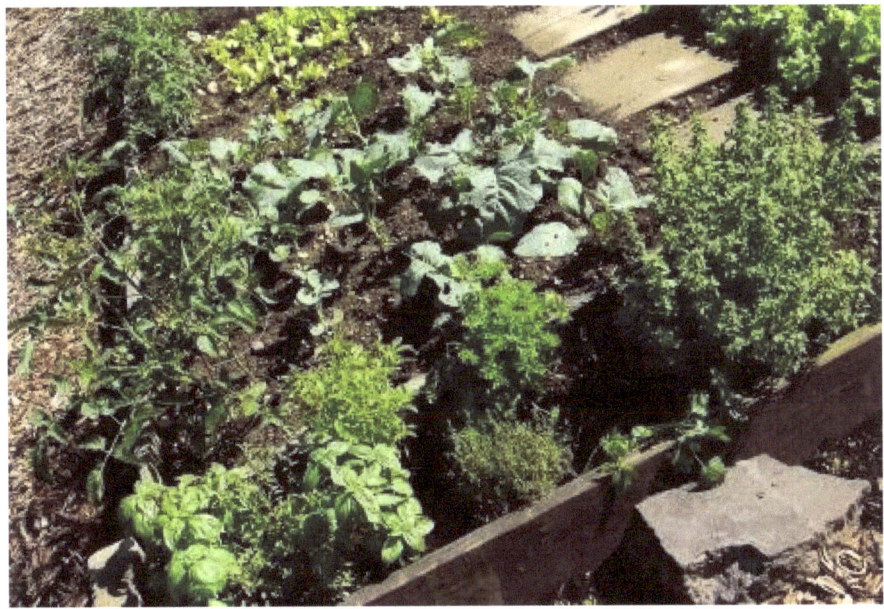

We are very fortunate today. We have access to so many herbs and spices, which were once available only at the local apothecary's. The wealth of the natural world is right here at our fingertips, and that is why this priceless natural heritage to keep us healthy should be well appreciated by one and all.

So look at all the benefits which you are going to get from these 30 commonly found herbs, spices, and plants, and plant them in your garden or in pots on your windowsill right now.

Remember much of this knowledge has been lost during the centuries, including the Alexandrian process with which Cleopatra kept her flowers fresh for months. Also, the industrial revolution and scientific progress made people leave their land and come to the cities.

So take your first step in using these herbs to heal and cure you naturally.

Cinnamon–Cinnamomum zeylanicum

Cinnamon is considered to be one of the most precious of spices, known to man since ancient times. Not only is it a very excellent addition to your cuisine, but it also is a natural healer.

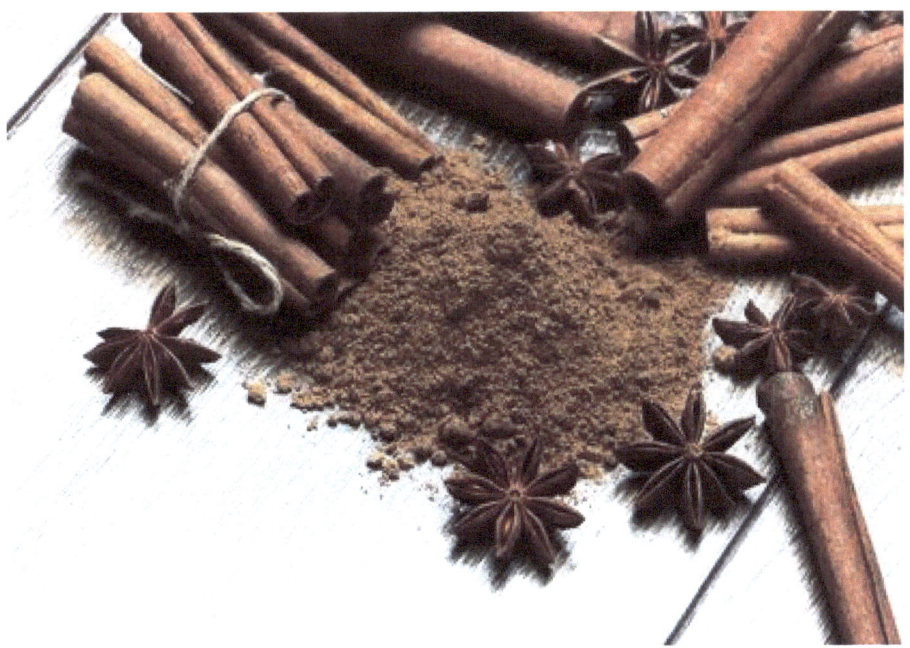

Cinnamon trees grow up to 15 to 18 m in height, in the wilderness, but when they are cultivated in plantations, they are chopped off close to the ground. This is so that the cultivators can get a fresh crop of shoots all the year around.

The shoots are harvested every two years, and the bark removed. When the bark is put out in the sun to dry, it curls up into quills. This is what you buy in the market.

The best cinnamon is grown in Sri Lanka. There is another associated plant, which is indigenous to China, and is called Cassia–Cinnamon cassia. It has almost the same properties as cinnamon, but it is bitter in taste, and is rough in feel and texture, when compared to original cinnamon.

The essential oil of the cinnamon is distilled from the broken bark. You can also get some oil from the leaves.

Cinnamon is excellent for poor circulation and colds. This is a best pick you up, especially when you want to feel warm. Ginger and cinnamon always go together, especially when they are put in warm drinks like milk and soup in the winters.

Cinnamon is milder than ginger, but it has a more powerful sustaining action.

When you are making a decoction with cinnamon, I would suggest using the quills, instead of using the powder. The powder makes the drink look muddy, and you need to filter it. Daily use of cinnamon in a glassful of hot milk made sure that I never suffered from cold feet and cold hands throughout the winter. Just add one little bit of cinnamon quill while boiling the milk with a little bit of ginger.

If you are suffering from a nose cold, all you have to do is pop a little bit of cinnamon in your mouth and keep chewing it.

Best Time-Tested Remedy for Colds

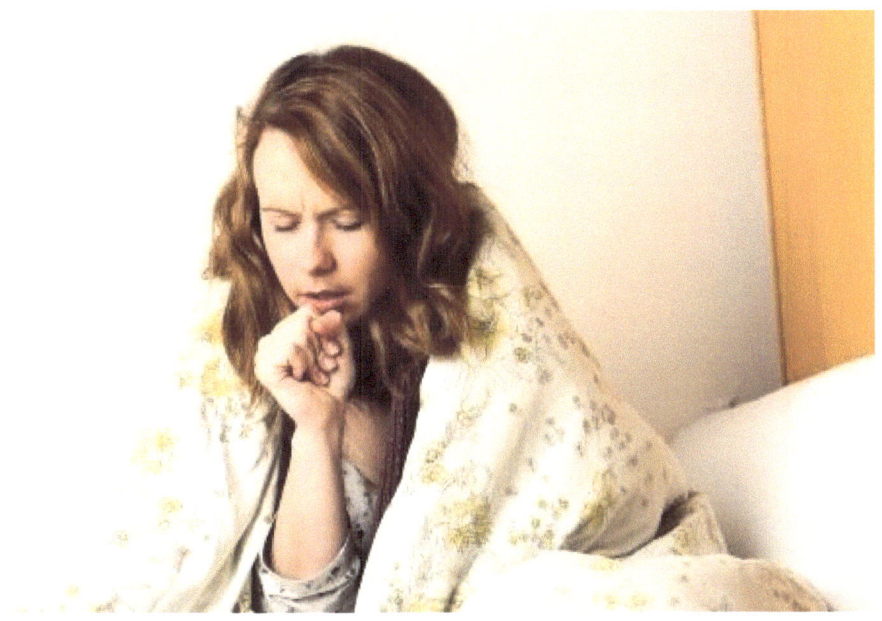

Just take **a glass of hot milk, add 2 teaspoons of powdered cinnamon, and a spoonful of honey. Then add a slug of brandy,** and go off to sleep.

Let me tell you this amusing story about cinnamon and brandy as experienced by yours truly. I do not drink. But my grandmother persuaded me, that Brandy was an excellent way in which I could keep the colds away, especially in the winter. So she used this remedy to treat me, because even though I was all grown up, I did not know much about grandmother's magic 3 tablespoons of brandy remedies, did I? The cold went away in about four days, but at every bedtime, I felt I was missing something. It was the brandy!

So unless you want to get addicted to the taste of milk, brandy, honey and cinnamon, use with care. But what a glorious way to get rid of colds!

Cinnamon is used in cuisine is an excellent flavoring for pork and chicken dishes. Baked foods and meats like roast pork, biscuits, apple pies, and cakes cannot do without a touch of cinnamon.

Children suffering from diarrhea can be given 1 teaspoon of cinnamon powder in a glass of warm milk.

In ancient Indian medicine, cinnamon is used to stimulate the system and promote the absorption of other herbs and spices.

Making a Ginger and Cinnamon Decoction

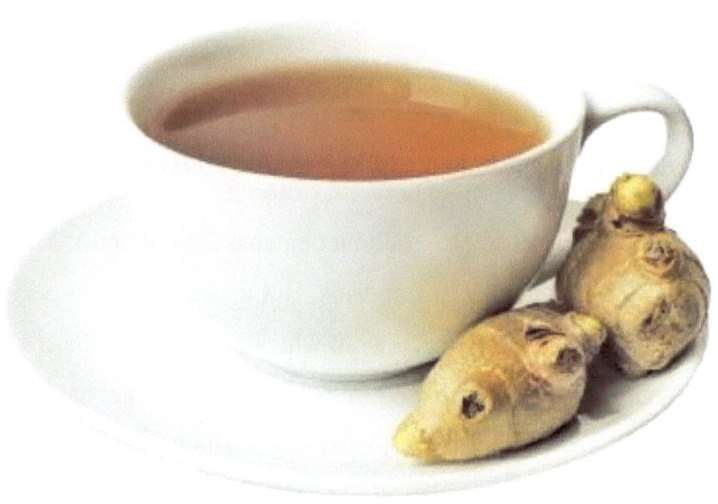

Try this remedy to get rid of colds. It is also excellent for keeping your mouth fresh and for curing infected gums and halitosis.

1 ½ sticks of broken cinnamon – about 7 inches all together.

1 inch of fresh ginger root, thinly sliced

half a cup of water.

1 teaspoon full of honey, if I am drinking it. I do not add the honey if I am using it as a mouthwash.

Simmer all the spices together, in a covered pan on low heat for about 10 minutes. Filter and drink hot.

Cayenne – Capsicum minimum

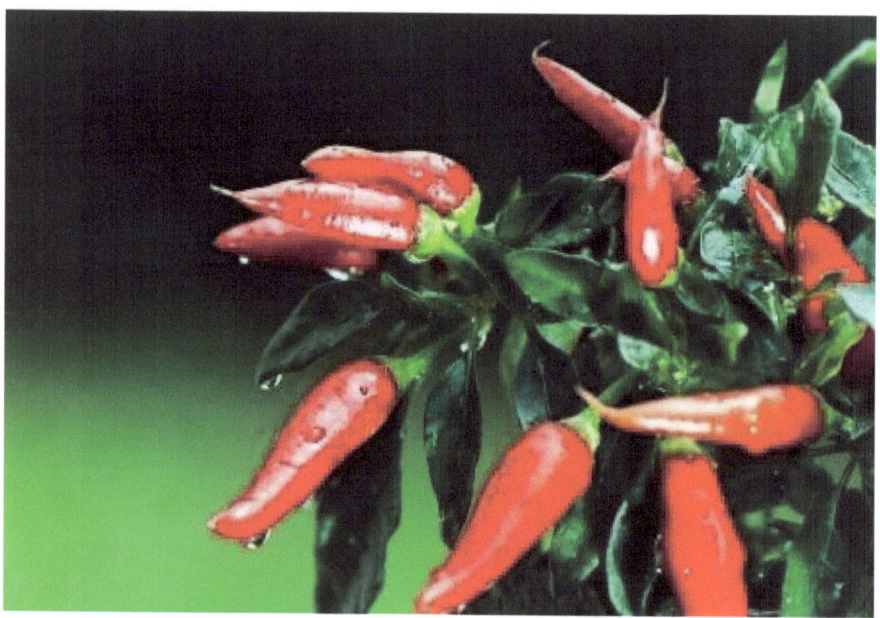

Cayenne powder, which you find in the market is definitely different from the vegetables you call capsicum or bell peppers. This Cayenne is better known as Chillies and is an herb/spice.

These hot chilies are natural stimulants, radiating heat throughout your whole body. It equalizes your body temperature from inside to your skin. That is why a pinch of cayenne is necessary to add warmth and heat to any soup which you are drinking in the winter.

Chilies are excellent for regulating your circulatory system, as well as strengthening your heart. Oil made from chilies are excellent to warm-up cold feet and cold hands and relaxing tense muscles.

Ancient and medieval herbalists assigned the chili to the sun, because it was hot. The effect was almost as if you had a small white hot sun radiating its seat and energy inside you. This effect can be equal to lying out in the sun, and feeling the warmth permeate through your heart, body and soul.

A pinch of this spice of life is going to add warmth to the dish, and help circulate its healing powers throughout your body.

In the 19th century, Cayenne was considered to be a very powerful stimulant. That is why it was used by herbalists extensively in small or in large doses to induce the metabolism to get activated naturally. Also, this helped in getting rid of all the toxic wastes accumulated in the body.

Cayenne is used as a tonic, antispasmodic, circulatory system stimulant and also a rubifacient.

Cayenne Hot Oil
Herbalists know all about the heating and the cooling power of different herbs and spices. So when do you use heating oils? If you are feeling too cold, stiff, chilled, and also, if some portions of your body are cold and stiff, especially in cases like arthritis, then you use a hot oil made up of cayenne. It is going to bring warmth to your body.

Make this right now for winter use, including chilblains, muscle aches, warming cold areas, improving circulation, spasms, and getting rid of chills from your bones.

Take these ingredients –

25 g cayenne pepper
2 inches ginger root

2 tablespoons mustard powder.

1/1 x 4 cups vegetable oil

2 teaspoons ground black pepper

Making an Infused Oil

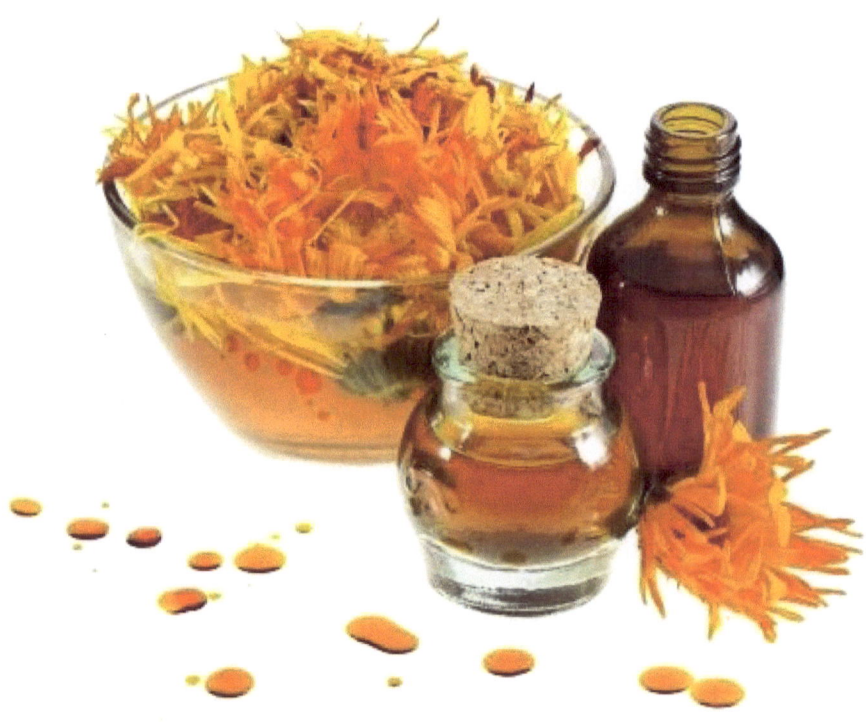

This infused oil has been made from Marigold Petals

Chop up the ginger root, and put half of the Cayenne pepper, black pepper and mustard powder, and all the oil into a container with a tight lid. Now place the container into a pan. Fill the pan up with water within 1 inch of the container's top, and simmer slowly for two hours. Thanks to this water bath, you are not going to worry about the oil burning and boiling.

Allow this mixture to cool. Filter it. Discard these herbs by putting them in your compost heap. Refill the oil canister with the remaining herbs and spices, and returned to the water, but. This is simmered gently for another two hours. Make sure that the water in the outer container is refilled so that it does not dry out.

Remember to filter it carefully and throw away any liquid which may have accumulated at the bottom. This residue is capable of spoiling the oil. Use this oil as often as possible, in very small quantities, because it is going to have a hot effect when placed in contact with your skin.

Lemon – Citrus lemonum

Once upon a time, lemons and oranges were considered to be so precious, that only the very rich could afford them. That is because they did not flourish in cold northern climates. So orange trees and lemon trees were grown in greenhouses and orangeries.

But nowadays we can use this versatile in all its forms – zest, peel, juice, oil, pips, and fruit, in one easily available package which can keep us healthy and fit and beautiful for long.

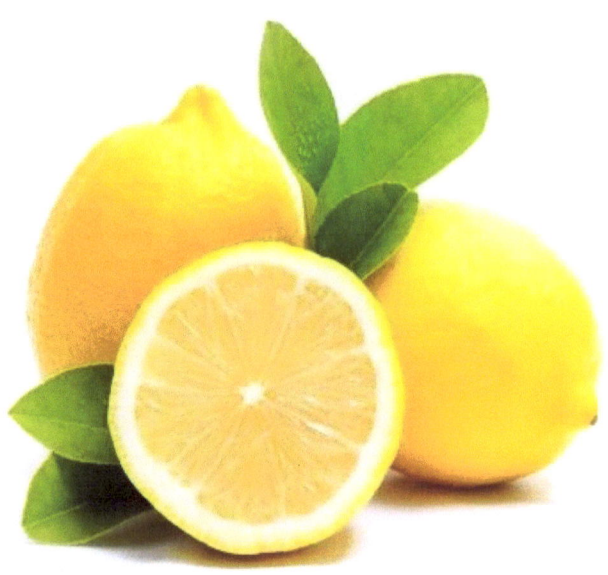

Lemon juice is refreshing and cooling. It has the sharp and clean taste that tones and detoxifies your system. Lemon and honey as a remedy for cold is just not an old wife's tale. It is a time-tested remedy.

Lemon for Fever

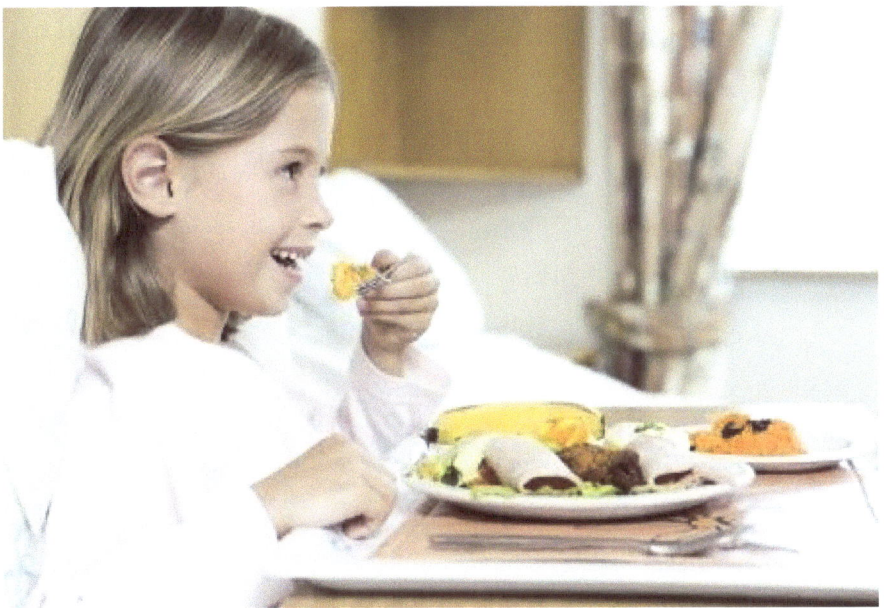

Add Lemon to the Diet of a Person Who Is Recuperating from Fever

If you are suffering from fever, use lemon as a diuretic to lower your temperature and get rid of all the accumulated infection and poisons in your body.

For this, you need the juice of one lemon in 2 and a half cups of water and 1 teaspoon of honey to taste. Drink as often as possible, because the more you drink it, the better your auto immune system is going to grow healthy.

Lemon Compress

Make a compress of the juice of one lemon in 5 cups of really cold water. This is excellent for reducing surface heat, and cooling down temperatures.

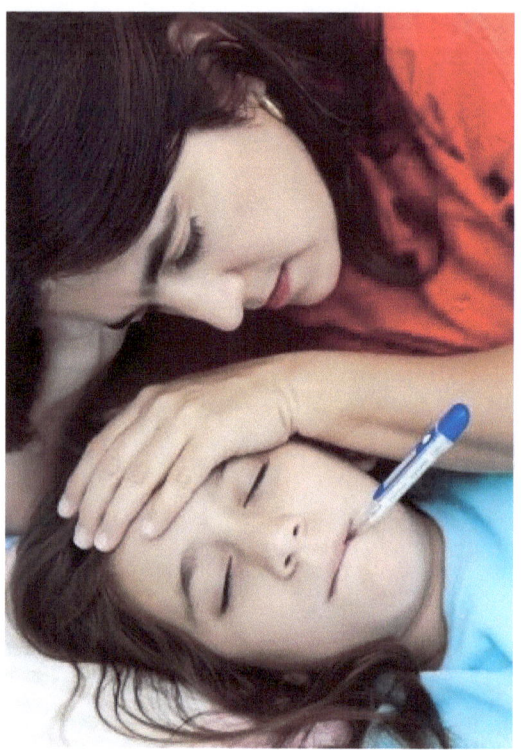

Lemon for Beauty and Health

Try adding a little bit of lemon juice into your bathing water. It is excellent as a refresher. Also, bed sheets soaked in lemon juice, especially after you are washing them off a fever bed is going to give your sheets nice and fresh and lemony smelling.

Skin Balm

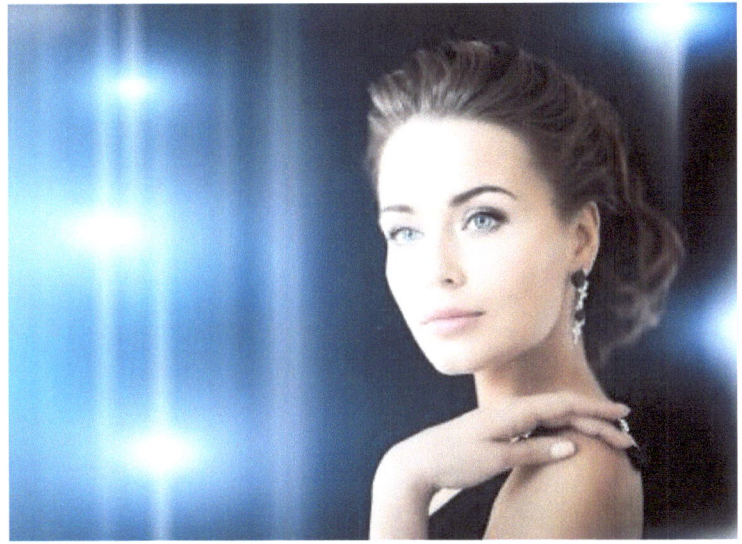

Make a lemon skin balm by mixing 40 spools of lemon juice with a peaceful full of almond oil. Add 2 teaspoons of clear honey. Mix them together, shake well and place in a glass bottle. This is extremely good for your skin, because it enriches and moisturizes it.

Lemon Body Lotion

You can also make lemon body lotions by mixing 1 ½ teaspoonful of water to the above skin balm recipe. Then smooth all over your body, after a shower. You may want to add a little bit of your favorite essential oil – not more than one drop, because these beauty preparations are not perfumed, except for the natural lemon fragrance.

Lemon is acid in the taste, but the moment you drink it, it will turn into an alkalizing agent. That is why if you are suffering from a lot of acidity in your body, you need to take lemon. This is also going to speed up the metabolism of your liver and digestive system.

Lemon juice and fresh water taken every morning, is an excellent way to start the day. It is also good for wadding off any potential infections. It is good to balance your nervous system, help to reduce HBP, maintain the vitality of your tissues and muscular system, and also is good for alleviating gout and rheumatism pains. Try it out if you are suffering from any of these ailments.

You can use the lemon oil directly by squeezing lemon peel and rubbing it directly over your skin. This is going to keep it healthy, blemish free, infection, free and smooth.

Ringworm and warts can also be cured by rubbing this antifungal, antiseptic and bactericidal skin all over the affected areas.

Cardamoms- Elettaria cardamomum

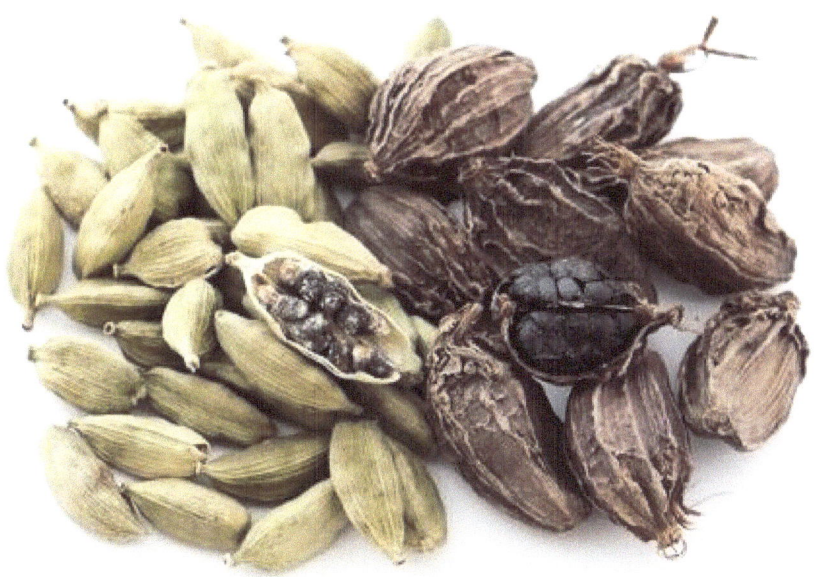

Cardamoms also belong to the ginger family, but their seeds are used as spices. There are two popular varieties of cardamoms available easily all over the world – green cardamoms and black cardamoms.

Cardamoms are natives of the southern portion of the Indian subcontinent, and Central America. The cardamoms are harvested, and dried in the sun, making sure that the seedpods do not split. In this manner, the powerful aromatic quality of the seeds is preserved until you need them.

You use these cardamoms by opening up the seedpods and crushing the seeds so that the aromatic qualities are released.

Cardamoms are not so powerful as ginger, so you can always use them, when you want a light and mild effect on your system and brain. Cardamoms, cloves and cinnamon are added to ginger and water to make refreshing teas, in the winter, to get your system toned.

Cardamoms are excellent for sinusitis, and you can chew them to get rid of cough and catarrh. At the same time you are sweetening your breath. So try adding cardamom seeds to milk, especially if you have a tendency towards chest infections.

For Caffeine Addicts

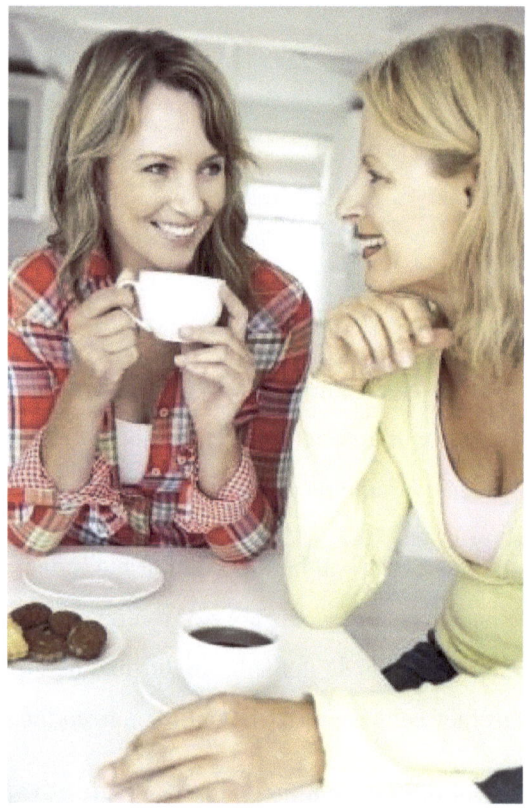

Can't Do without My Brew

In fact, if you are a caffeine addict, try adding some cardamoms to your daily brew of Java to neutralize that affect which may be occasionally over stimulating to your brain.

Mind Clearing Potpourri

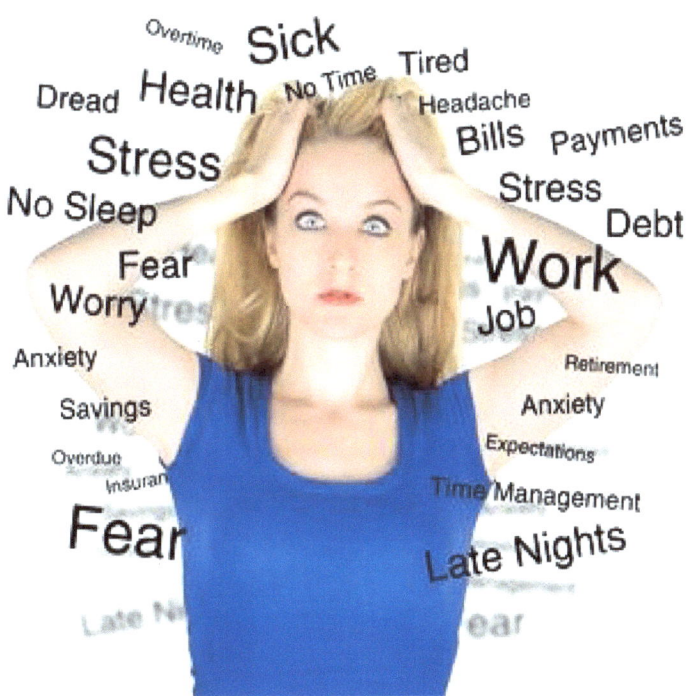

Are you suffering from an overloaded brain, which makes you lose your concentration, especially when you are working? Try this mind clearing spice and herbal mixture, which is amazingly good and effective. Just put it in a glass bottle and place it on your desk. And take a hearty sniff, whenever you think you need to concentrate on something. Just one whiff, and it is going to calm your anxiety, promote mental clarity and alertness and make you relax, especially if you are stressed out.

Take 2 teaspoons each of **powdered cloves, cardamom, cinnamon, sea salt and rosemary**. Add the **zest of one lemon**. Add just enough of **brandy** to make in a smooth paste. I normally do this by grinding all the spices together, and then put them in my glass bottle. Then I stir in the brandy and put on the air tight lid. Beats smelling salts any day!

Onions –Allium cepa

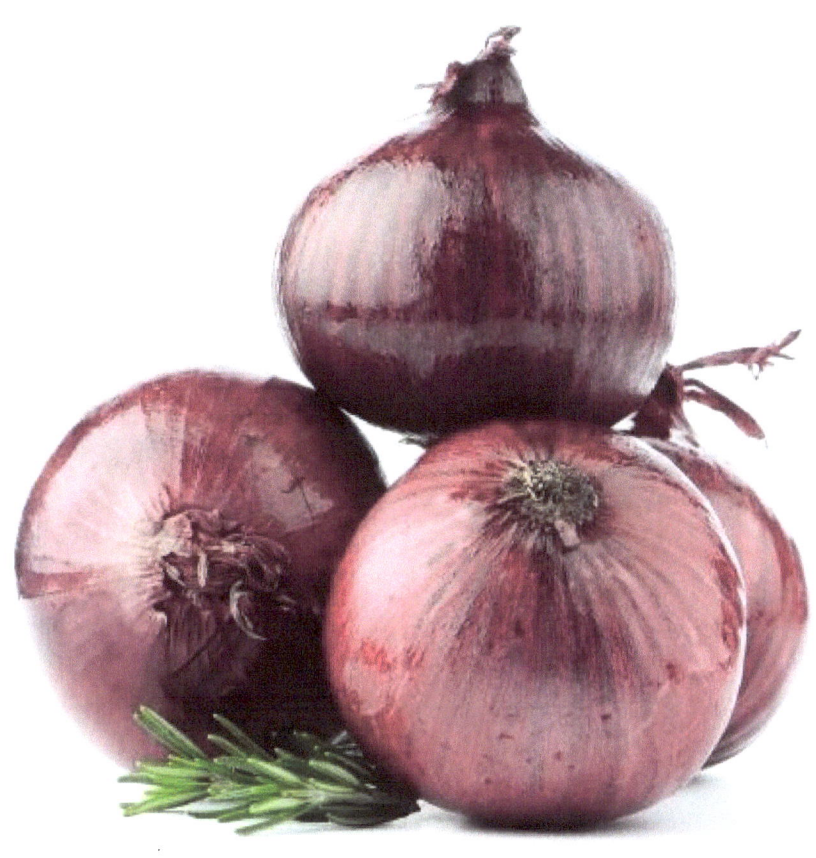

Onions also have excellent curative powers because they are also antiallergic, antiparasitic, antifungal, antibacterial, antiseptic and antiviral. When you feel garlic to be too strong, you can use onions, because this has a more soothing effect. This is definitely more suitable for children, old people, and people who are prone to bacterial and viral infections.

Onion milk

Believe it or not, I have seen people drinking milk in which onions have been boiled. I normally add honey and cinnamon to milk, but this medicinal milk is more of a health giving drink rather than the normal milk we have for breakfast.

So if you are intolerant to natural milk, you can also try soy milk, which is equally healthy and beneficial, though of course not the perfect substitute for the real stuff.

Slice up one small onion, and boil it in 2 ½ cups of milk. Simmer on low heat for another 20 minutes, until all the essential oils of the onions have been incorporated in the milk. Filtered this milk and use the onions in your cooking. Add a pinch of cinnamon, and some honey, just for taste, if you are drinking it.

You can refrigerate it for a couple of days in the refrigerator. You can give this as often as possible to children over seven years. For babies, you just rub three drops on the feet and the chest to prevent chest infections and congestion. For children less than six years, give them 1 teaspoon of this healthy medicinal milk, up to six times a day.

See them remain healthy and fit!

The juice of the onion has been used since ancient times for curing infections, burns, and spots.

In fact, onion juice was applied on scalds and burns to take away the heat. That is because it is an excellent antifungal, so the next time you find yourself slightly burned in a kitchen accident, just put that burned portion under the water, while you chop up an onion with your other hand. Apply on the affected region and cover with a bandage.

Onion Poultice

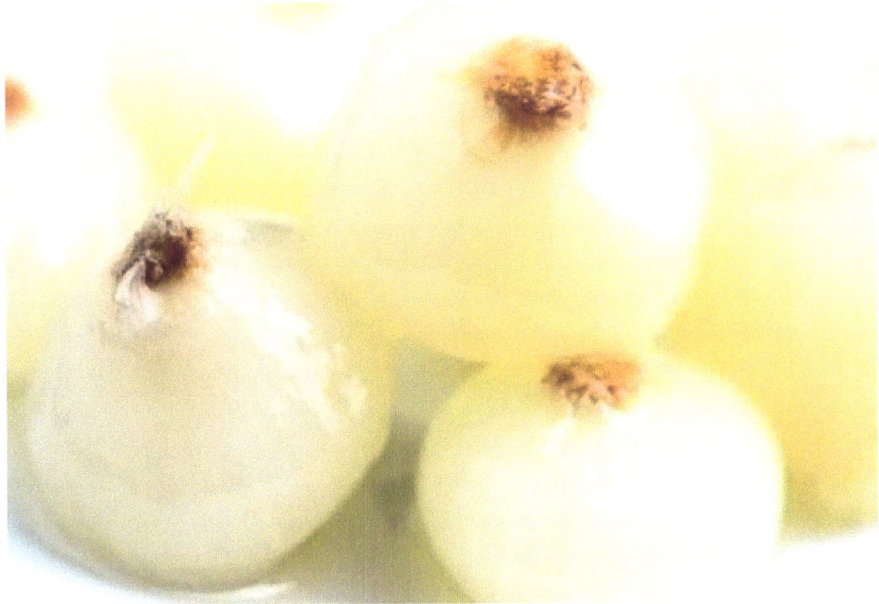

An onion poultice is excellent for relieving earache. In Victorian times, a whole onion was roasted until it was soft. It was then cut into half, and applied to the affected area, with a bandage. This warm fomentation soon took the earache away. You can also use this roasted onion to clean wounds and prevent infections.

For all those people who find onion and garlic too strong for their Constitution, try the leek and also shallots, which belong to the same family, but are milder in comparison. Leek soup is excellent for people living in cold climates. In ancient times, this was also considered to be an excellent way to prevent and heal pneumonia and chronic cough, especially in continuous damp and cold weather.

Traditional Soups

http://www.marthastewart.com/867269/traditional-french-onion-soup

http://www.greatbritishkitchen.co.uk/recipebook/index.php?option=com_ra pidrecipe&page=viewrecipe&recipe_id=1145

Garlic– Allium sativum

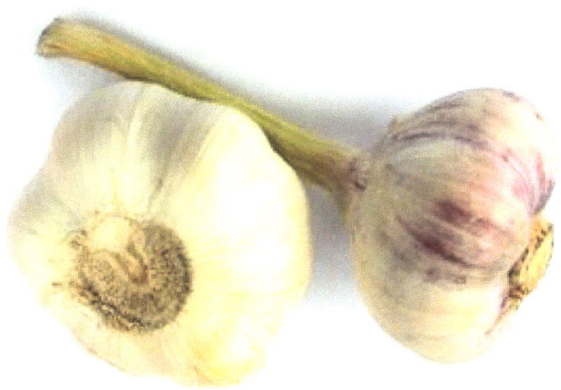

Garlic is a perennial herb with decorative flowers and long leaves. The garlic bulb was put into use, and it consists of several cloves, each covered by a skin. The bulb itself is covered by a white fragile membranous skin.

Garlic is antifungal, anti-septic, expectorant, antibacterial, antiviral, and also a stimulant for your circulatory system. Nicholas Culpeper, one of the most famous of medieval herbalists caused this the poor man's treacle, because it has the power to cure all hurts and diseases. You may almost say that no other plant has so many beneficial qualities, and much of its properties are exaggeration, but scientific research has proven garlic to "deliver the goods", each time every time, and without fail.

Garlic originated in Central Asia, from where it spread all over the world. In ancient times, it was used to prevent and heal infections and contain contagion. In countries where people suffer from cholera and typhus regularly, garlic is eaten in every meal as a preventative.

Even though garlic is an essential part of the cuisine of lots of countries, many people do not eat garlic because they consider it to be strong smelling. In the same manner, they do not eat onions, because of the sulfur content.

It is the strong and offensive aroma of garlic is what is going to cure your chest of infections, and its therapeutic activity is enhanced by these natural products.

So if you want to buy them in tablet form, pearl form, or in liquid form, just because you do not like the smell, remember fresh garlic's the best option for you.

Make this garlic, easily digestible, by roasting it. Try mixing it up with garlic bread and garlic butter.

Garlic Bread and Garlic Butter

http://www.wikihow.com/Make-Garlic-Bread

This is the way which you can get your daily intake of garlic butter, as well as garlic bread. Powdered garlic is also an excellent addition to spicy salts.

Garlic is considered to be an excellent way in which you can lower your cholesterol level, as well as your blood sugar. Chest infections are never going to attack a person who eats plenty of garlic.

Garlic Rub

Also, you can make garlic rubs – add half a teaspoonful of ginger powder and three cloves of garlic to half a cup of coconut or mustard oil. Allow to boil. Let cool and then apply gently over the chest, to prevent congestion and facilitate breathing. Do not try this on babies. For children, reduce the quantities to one clove of garlic, and three pinches of ginger powder to half a cup of mild coconut oil, or almond oil.

Cloves – Eugenia Aromatica

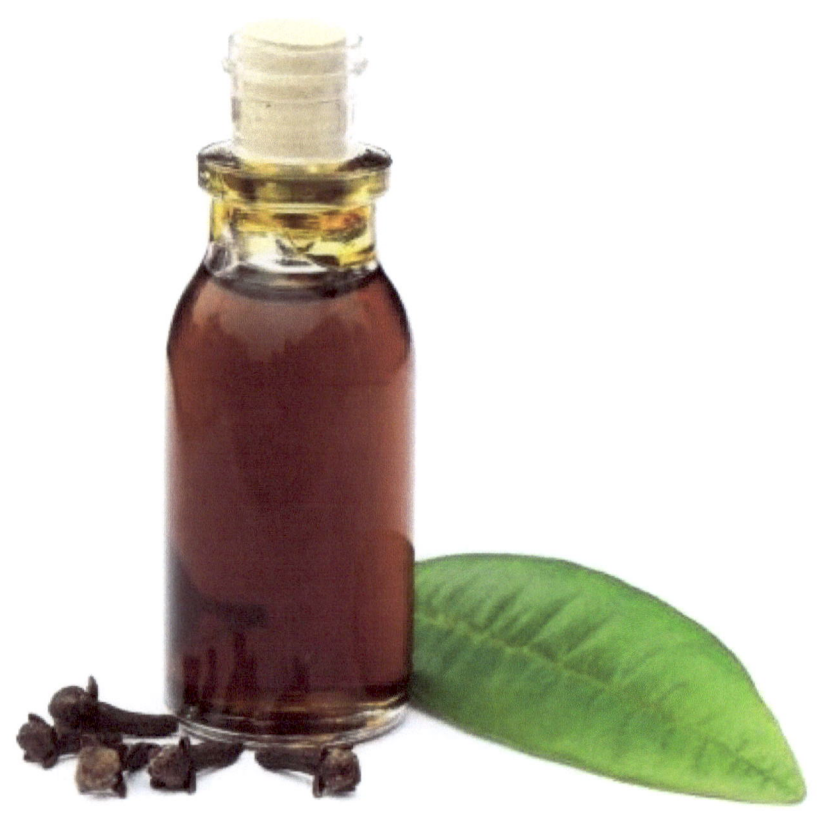

The deep and distinct smell of cloves are enough to reassure the body and the mind, and raise your spirits. In ancient Chinese writing, more than 5000 years ago, there have been references to cloves. These are the buds of a tall tree native to Indonesia, discovered in the 15th century by the Portuguese. But in the East, cloves were already been in use for millenniums, where they grew it locally. 15th century Europe went to war for getting control over these Indonesian islands, and it was only to the 18th century, when seedlings were smuggled out from Indonesia that the French established plantations in Zanzibar.

The moment you hear the term clove oil, your immediate response is – excellent for toothache. Just soak a small wad of cotton wool in the oil. Hold that against the infected tooth. The anesthetic quality of this powerful oil is going to bring immediate relief. Do not apply directly on your skin, because it is very powerful. It is going to cause blisters on your gums and in your mouth.

People suffering from bronchial infections can add three cloves to any herbal infusion or decoction which they are concocting. Toothache and oral hygiene is well served with a mouthwash made up of six cloves in half a cup of water, boiled and cooled. Rinse your mouth out with this mouthwash regularly after brushing your teeth. You get a natural breath freshener, as well as a powerful antiseptic mouthwash all in one.

Analgesic Rub for Headache and Backache
Take 25 g of ground cloves
50 g of grated fresh ginger root, Rosemary and Sage
4 teaspoons cayenne pepper
100 grams of thyme.
2 ½ cups vegetable oil

This is excellent, especially if you are suffering from backache and headache. Make an infused oil, as instructed above. Just apply it all over the affected area, and let the cloves work their magic.

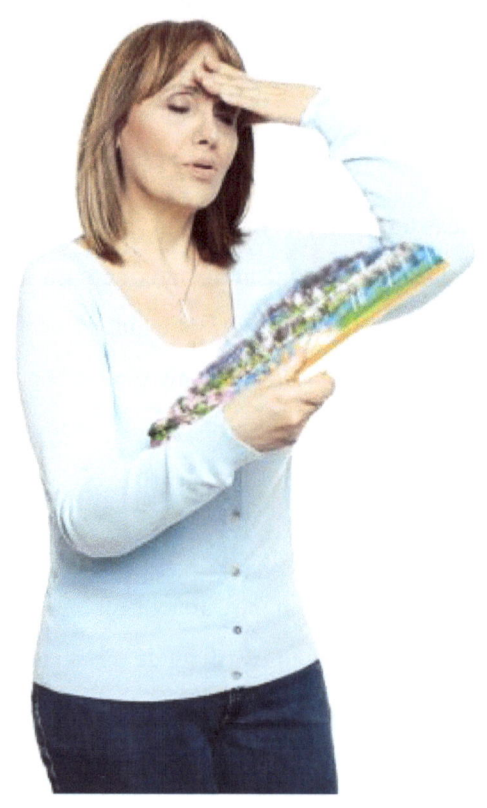

Tension and Stress Can Cause Headaches

Cloves are extremely powerful germicidal, antibacterial, antiviral and antifungal spices. Historical legend says that when the Dutch knowing that their monopoly over the clove islands in Indonesia had been taken over by other Europeans, destroyed the plantations of these trees in an island, it was overtaken with previously unknown epidemics and destroyed. The cloves protected the people of that land from alien bacteria and viruses.

Fennel- Foeniculum Vulgare

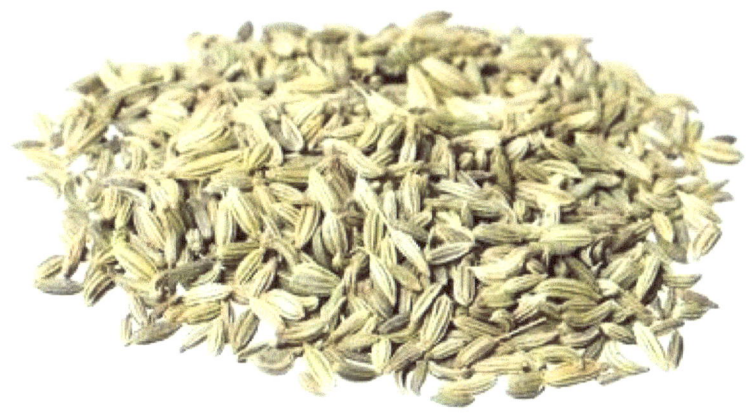

Believe it or not, the ancient Greeks used Fennel seeds to reduce weight. It is Carminative and digestive properties have already been well-documented through millenniums. No Eastern meal is considered to be complete, without a spoonful of fennel, followed up with some rock candy. This is to help digest that heavy meal you just had a little while ago.

In medieval times, when fasting was a way of life, wise women used a pound of garlic, pepper and peony seeds, along with fennel seeds, taken often, so that they did not feel really hungry. This is because chewing the seeds calmed the stomach and stayed the tangs of hunger.

Nursing mothers in the East, take fennel tea every day, so that their children do not suffer from colic. Also, if your baby is suffering from colic problems, just give him a teaspoonful of this fennel seed tea. It is going to relieve the wind.

Fennel as a Diuretic

Fennel is excellent as a diuretic. It prevents water retention. So just drink it as a tea, or just eat the seeds as often as you can. Also, if you are suffering from arthritis, just try adding fennel seed to your daily diet. You are soon going to see an improvement.

How to Make Herbal Teas

For all those people interested in how to make herbal teas, here is a good link.

http://www.countryliving.com/cooking/about-food/herbal-teas-0906_2

Drinking this fennel herbal tea regularly is considered to be excellent for eyesight. You can also use this tea as an eyewash for tired, inflamed and sore eyes.

Tip-milk is rarely added to herbal teas. That is because it suppresses the flavor of the original herbal tea. However, if you do want to use milk, remember to pour the milk first in your cup, and then stir in the infused tea. This will prevent the milk from scalding. You may want to add lemon juice, honey, and even cayenne pepper, depending on whether you are drinking this tea to warm, cool, or just enjoy natural herbs.

Honey in Basil and Sage tea is excellent to soothe an infected throat. Cayenne in Sage tea is excellent for breaking fevers.

"Smoking" Fennel Seeds

The Native Americans use steam, smoke and burnt herbs, to relax patients in sweat lodges and also in purification rituals. Burning seeds, especially for fumigation is a tradition which has come down through the ages.

The ancient Anglo-Saxons took fennel, dried rushes/grass and cotton, and set them on fire. Then they fumigated their homes with this smoke.

Fennel is an excellent seed which can be smoked, by burning them in a charcoal holder. Then inhale the smoke deeply. This relaxes your body and de – stresses your mind.

Parsley

Someone once asked me whether Parsley and coriander were the same. And then where did cilantro come into the equation? And then there was something called Mexican Culantro. Well, this was confusing.

Parsley and coriander rather look similar, especially the leaves. But just break off a Parsley leaf, and inhale deeply. The aromatic oil is unforgettable and different from coriander. Once smelt, never forgotten.

So for all those people who are confused between parsley, cilantro, coriander, coriander is cilantro – different names for East and West. Culantro is another plant family altogether. Parsley belongs to the same family as coriander, but it is more aromatic, and has longer stems.

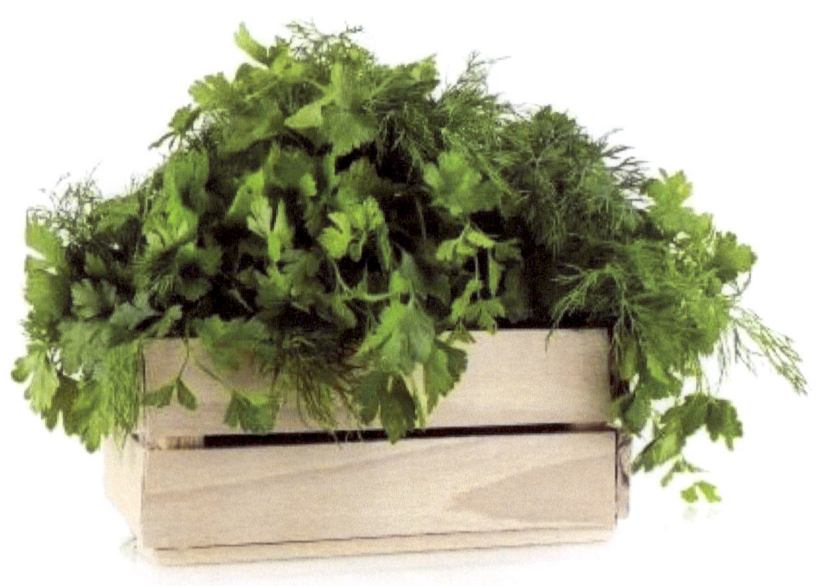

Parsley is excellent in cuisine, especially when eaten with meat and fish. This is useful for bladder, kidney, as well as urinary infections.

It has antiseptic, diuretic, digestive, carminative and tonic qualities.

Parsley root has been used in ancient Chinese medicine, as well as in Egyptian Greek and other ancient medicines, to keep them healthy. In fact Parsley is considered to be a woman's Herb. Parsley root and Parsley seeds are definitely not advised to women when they are expecting.

In the First World War, Parsley tea was used extensively to cure men, especially when they were suffering from kidney complications brought on through infection and dysentery. Also, Parsley poultices made up of freshly ground leaves and stems, were applied on skin, especially to get rid of eruptions and spots.

Parsley is recommended to women who are reaching menopause. That is because the leaves maintain the balance of the body's hormones.

Healthy Parsley Soup

This is a traditional soup in which Parsley has been used to promote good health in young women and old women.

3 tablespoons butter

One onion, whole

6 tablespoons flour

2 ½ cups milk

1 cup water

1 teaspoon salt

100 grams fresh parsley, finely chopped

Half cup light cream

Two egg yolks

This is a French traditional soup, which is made by melting the butter and adding the milk, water, onion, flour and salt. Simmer on low heat, after you have brought it to the boil for one hour.

Remove the onion. Add the cream, and beaten egg yolks. Cook gently without boiling, until the soup is thick. Add the parsley, just before serving. Serve at once.

You may also want to add garlic croutons, as an extra garnish if you want.

This is excellent for women were suffering from PMT, stress, headache and cramps, by toning up your circulatory and natural system.

Rosemary

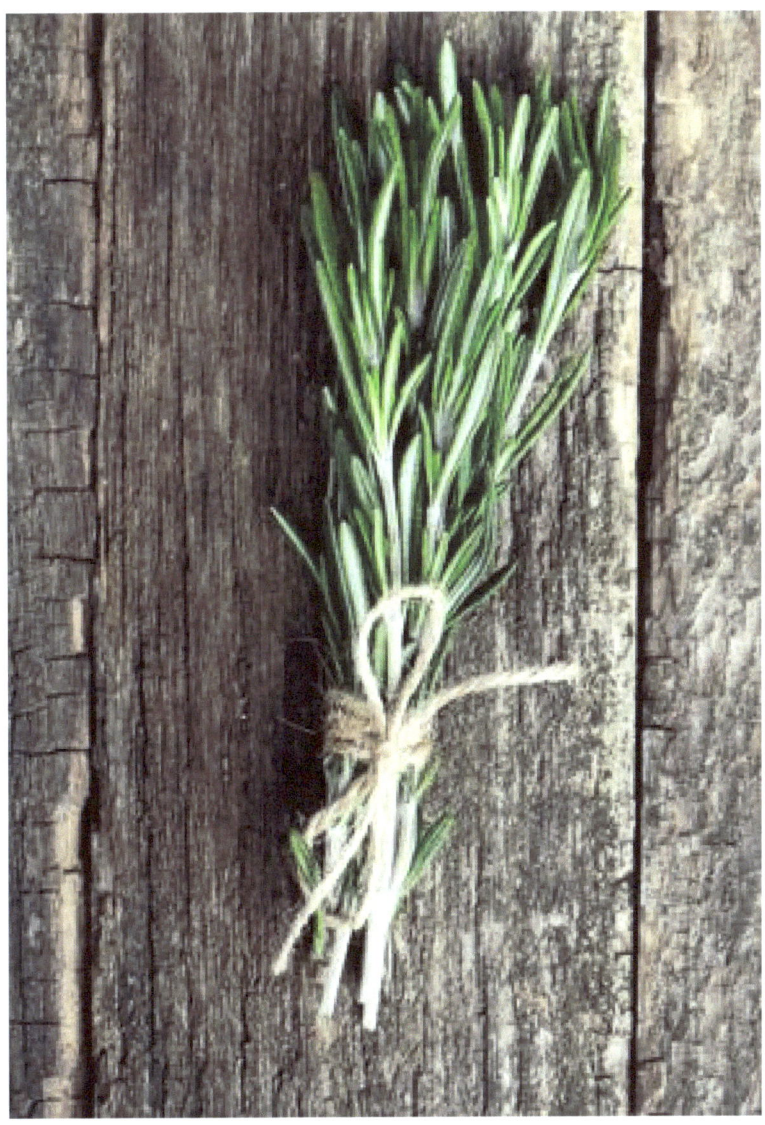

Are you going to Scarborough Fair? Parsley, sage, rosemary, and thyme.

Remember me to one who lives there, she once was a true love of mine.

[Traditional song made popular by Simon and Garfunkel]

Rosemary has long been known by herbalists, and physicians as one of the most important herbs to heal and to cure, as well as in cuisine and remedies. In fact, 16th-century herbal books spoke about sprinkle rosemary leaves among your clothes, and you are not going to suffer from moths. And the rosemary flowers were distilled with other spices to make an excellent breath freshener in those days of yore.

Making a Rosemary Tincture

But as I do not have distilled water of rosemary flowers, I am going to collect the other ingredients of this recipe – a few cloves, mace, cinnamon, and he seed and rosemary flowers and leaves. After that, I am going to make a tincture by mixing 25 g of these dried herbs/spices and 2 ½ cup of alcoholic liquid. The dosage of tinctures are small yet effective. These are allowed to sleep and infused, and the tincture gets more powerful with the passing of time.

This was normally done in ancient times by boiling the Herb and spices in wine. Tinctures are normally used in very small quantities, so take a small dose, according to that suggested by your herbal advisor, depending on your ailment.

People who do not drink alcohol are going to dilute the dose in ¼ cup water. I leave this uncovered for several hours, while the alcohol evaporates.

When I use this as a Rosemary gargle and mouthwash, I use just 2 teaspoons in a glassful of water with which to swish my mouth.

This evergreen shrub flowers in early spring or late winter. The tonic is classic and better, and considered to be an improving Herb for your digestion and your liver. A small glass of Rosemary wine was used as an aperitif, half an hour before one took a heavy meal, so that the digestive system got ready for future action.

Rosemary Conditioner

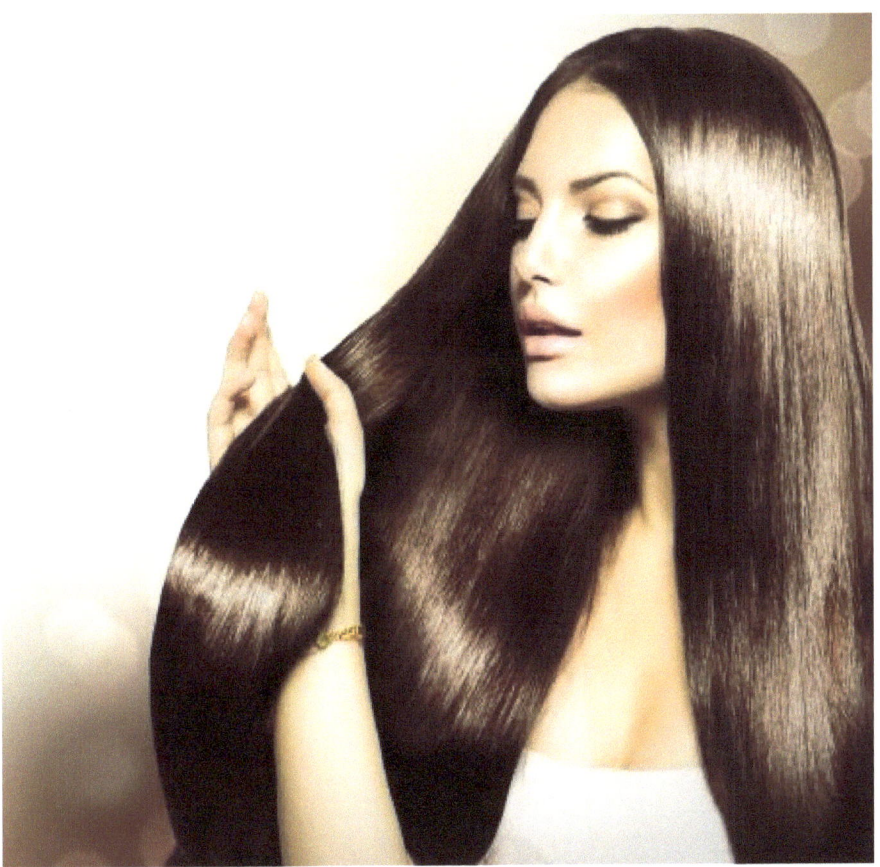

Rosemary is excellent for beauty, especially as a hair tonic. Add 2 fistfuls of rosemary to coconut oil, and allow to cook in the sun for about two weeks. This is the slow cooking method. But if you are in a hurry, you may also want to boil these leaves, for two hours – infused oils –, removing the rosemary leaves, filtering the coconut oil, and then going back to the next round of rosemary leaf infusion. You have very precious rosemary essential infused oil.

Or you can try this method – take 30 g of fresh rosemary leaves, and 150 mL of coconut oil. Infused over a bain marie for two hours, then strain. This conditioner can be made stronger by repeating up to three times with fresh rosemary leaves.

Apply straight on your hair after you have had a shampoo. You do not need any other conditioner. That is, if you prefer the coconut smell and untangled hair. I normally rub this well straight into my scalp, about 30 minutes before shampooing. Then I wash my hair normally.

Conclusion

These are just some of the herbs, spices and plants, which help keep you healthy and beautiful. So bless the bounty of nature, and take full advantage of all the benefits that she has given to us. We should be thankful to all those ancients who took the trouble of experimenting with different herbs and spices, and wrote down their unique qualities to heal and cure suffering mankind.

Many of these herbs and spices are very easily available in your garden, or in the market today, so live long and prosper with natural herbs and their bounty.

Author Bio

Dueep Jyot Singh is a Management and IT Professional who managed to gather Postgraduate qualifications in Management and English and Degrees in Science, French and Education while pursuing different enjoyable career options like being an hospital administrator, IT,SEO and HRD Database Manager/ trainer, movie scriptwriter, theatre artiste and public speaker, lecturer in French, Marketing and Advertising, ex-Editor of Hearts On Fire (now known as Solstice) Books Missouri USA, advice columnist and cartoonist, publisher and Aviation School trainer, ex- moderator on Medico.in, banker, student councilor ,travelogue writer … among other things! One fine morning, she decided that she had enough of killing herself by Degrees and went back to her first love -- writing. It's more enjoyable! She already has 48 published academic and 14 fiction- in- different- genre books under her belt.

When she is not designing websites or making Graphic design illustrations for clients , she is browsing through old bookshops hunting for treasures, of which she has an enviable collection – including R.L. Stevenson, O.Henry, Dornford Yates, Maurice Walsh, C.N.Williamson, Sapper, Bartimeus and the crown of her collection- Dickens "The Old Curiosity Shop," and so on… Just call her "Renaissance Woman") - collecting herbal remedies, acting like Universal Helping Hand/Agony Aunt, or escaping to her dear mountains for a bit of exploring, collecting herbs and plants and trekking.

Check out some of the other JD-Biz Publishing books

Health Learning Series

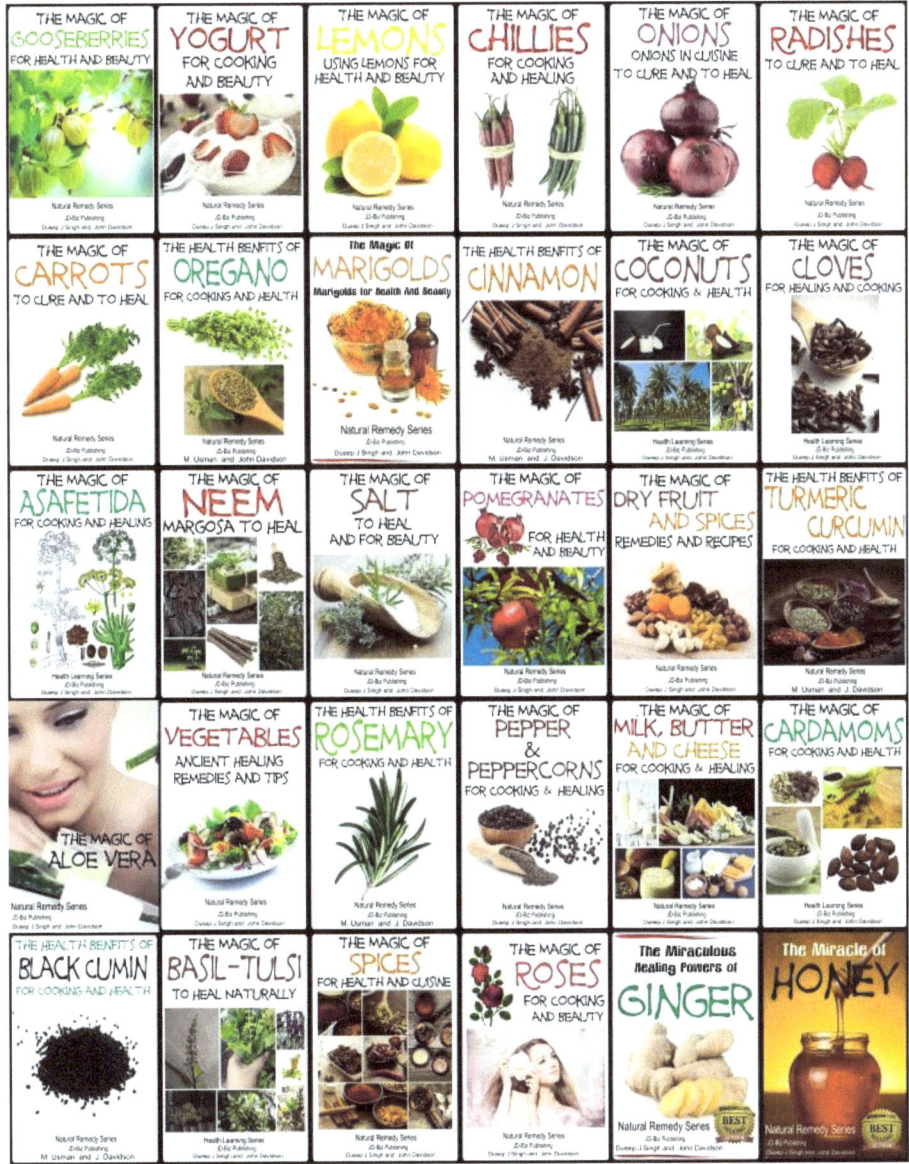

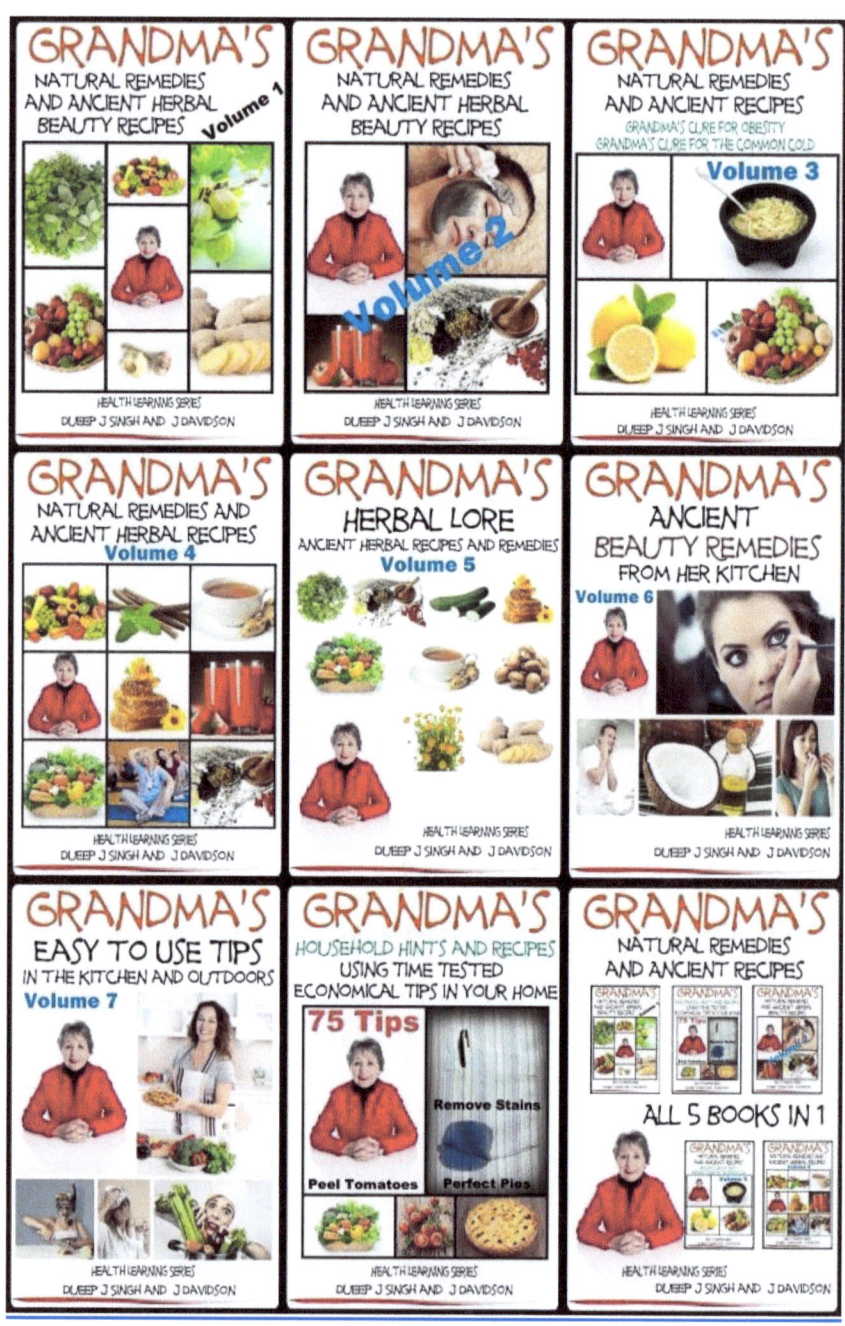

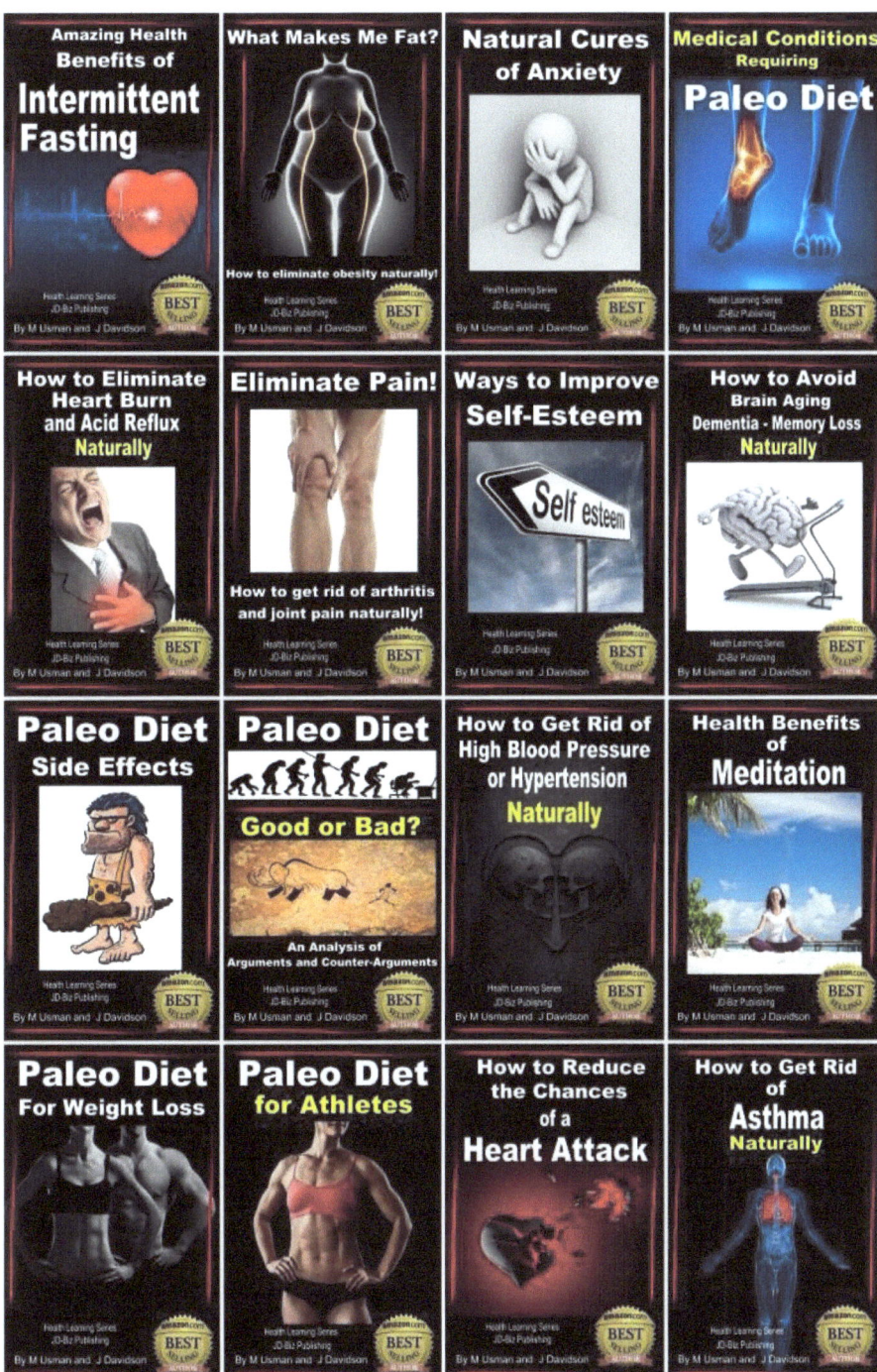

Amazing Animal Book Series

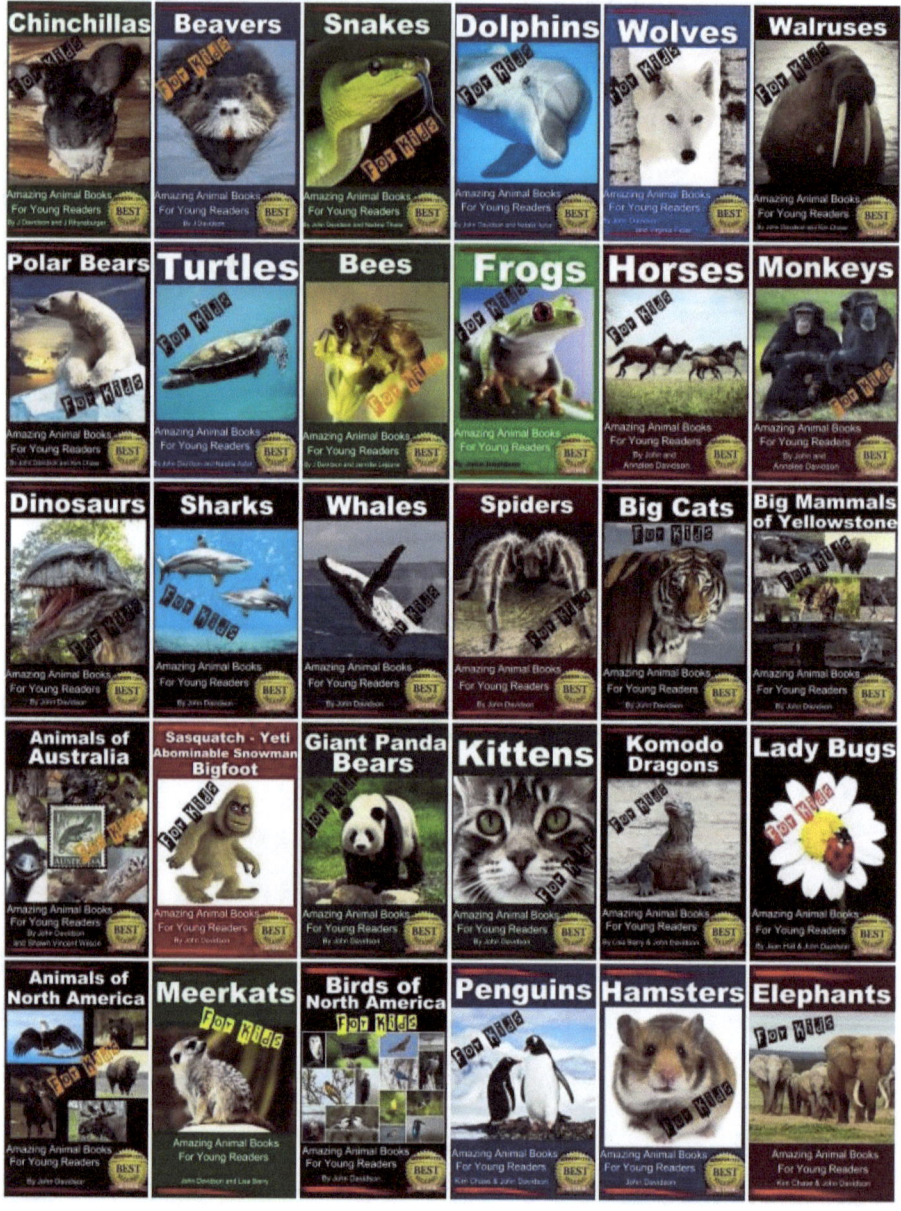

Learn To Draw Series

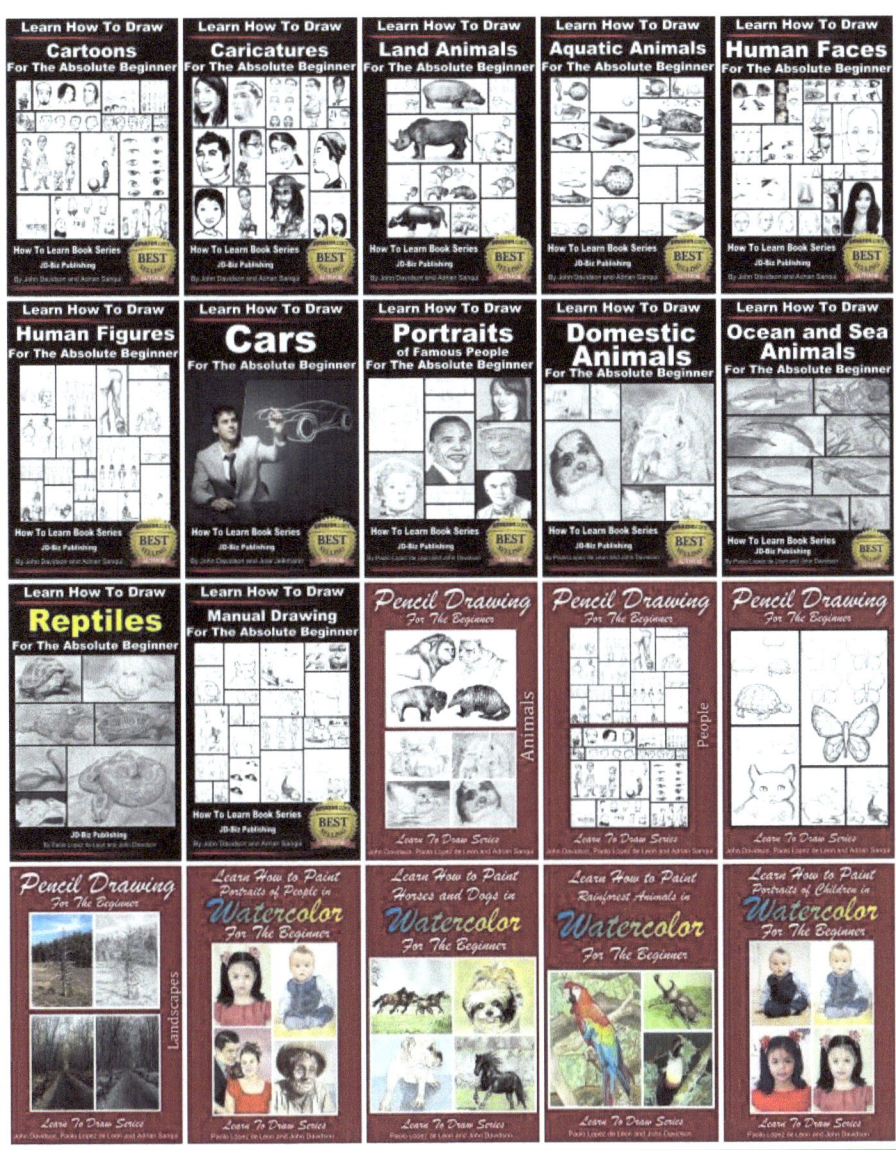

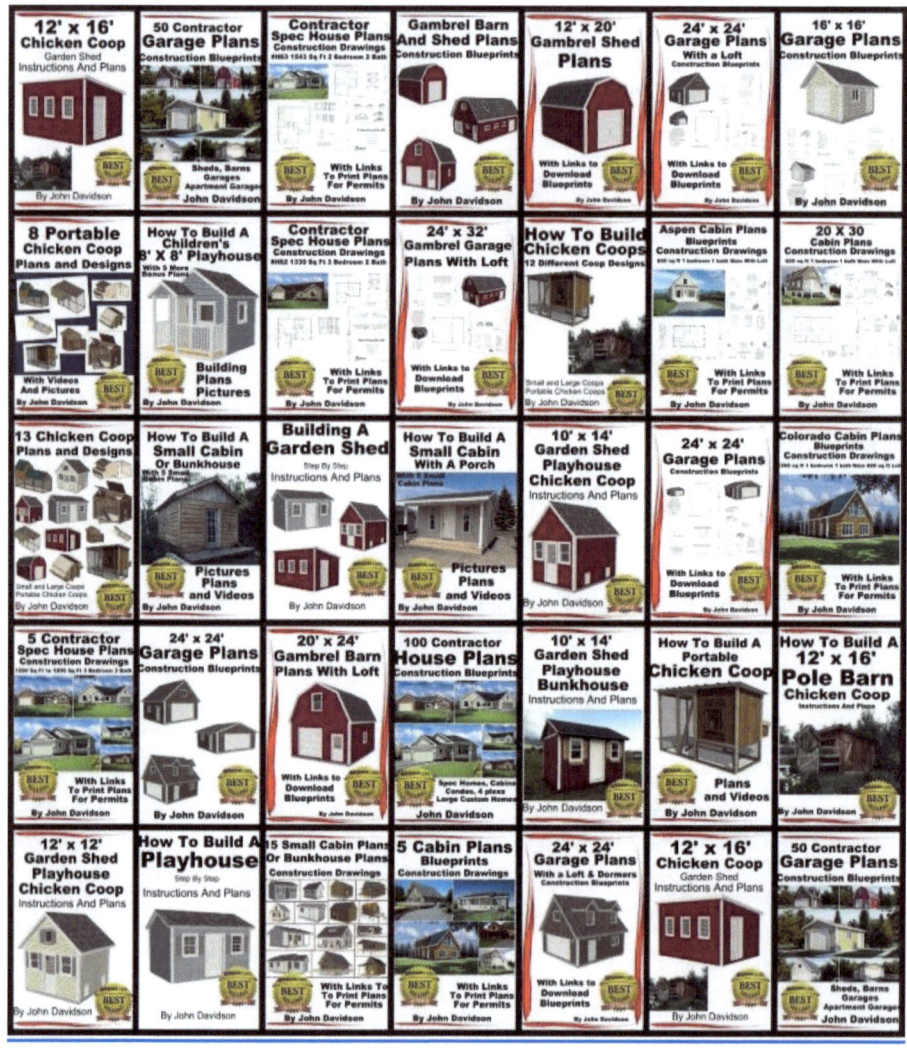

Entrepreneur Book Series

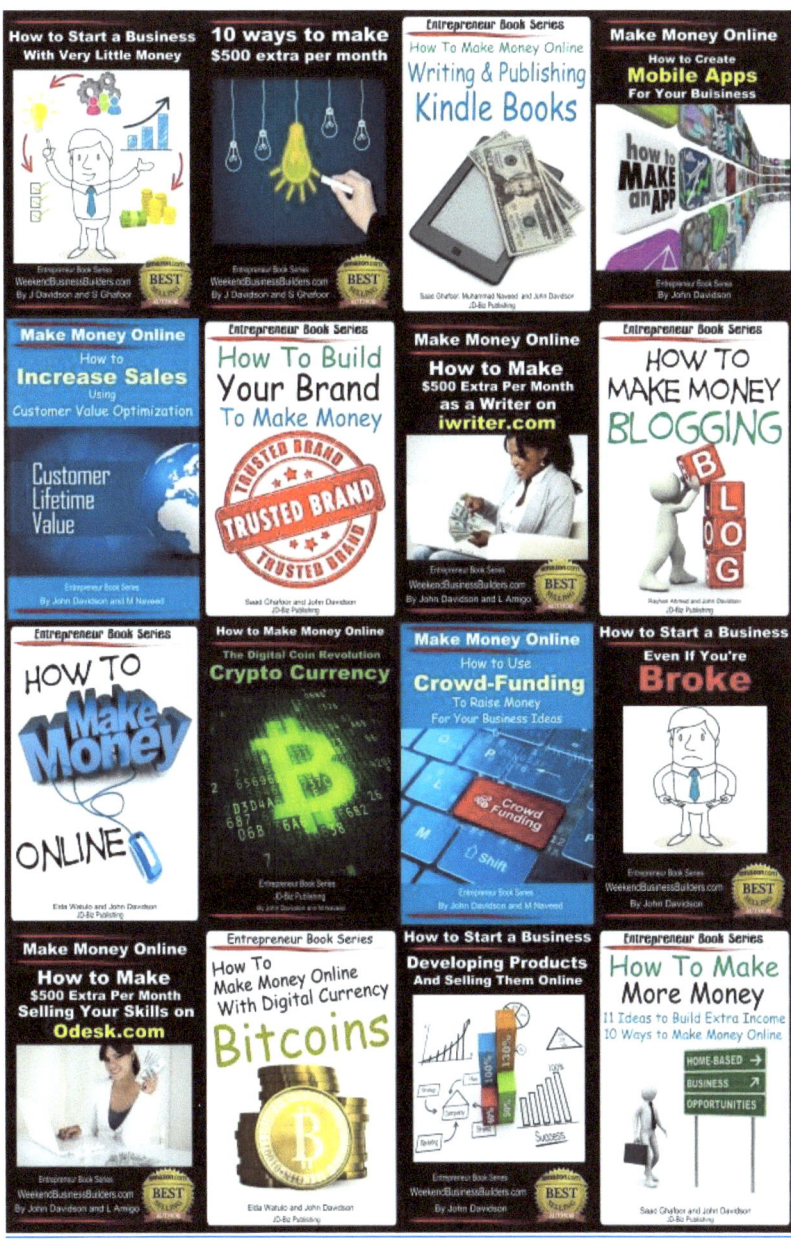

Our books are available at

1. Amazon.com

2. Barnes and Noble

3. Itunes

4. Kobo

5. Smashwords

6. Google Play Books

Download Free Books!

http://MendonCottageBooks.com

Publisher

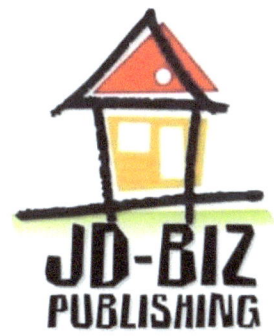

JD-Biz Corp

P O Box 374

Mendon, Utah 84325

http://www.jd-biz.com/

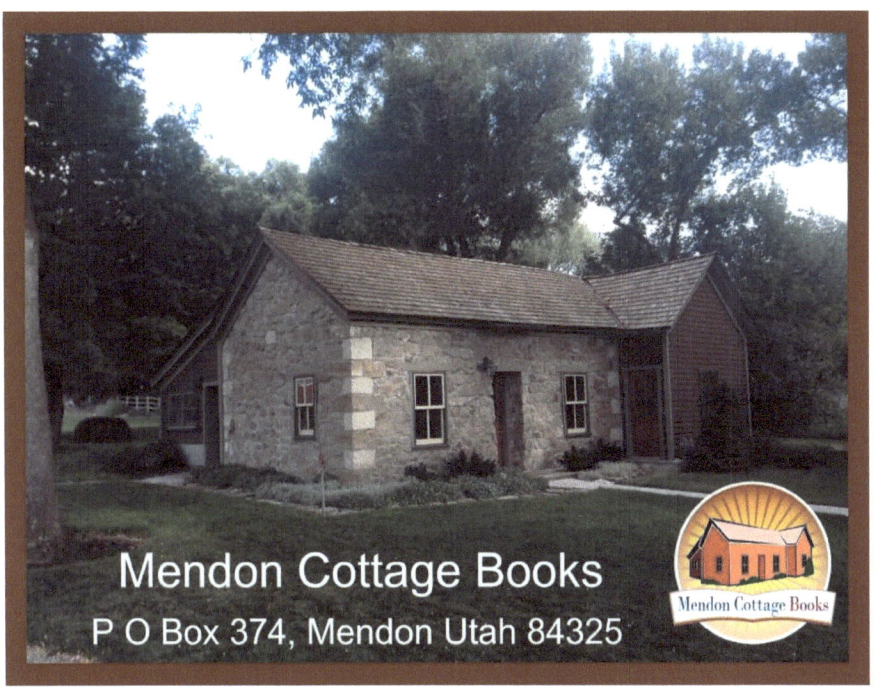

Mendon Cottage Books

P O Box 374, Mendon Utah 84325

www.ingramcontent.com/pod-product-compliance
Lightning Source LLC
Chambersburg PA
CBHW050824290526
45792CB00001B/247